Dedication

For all my fellow psoriasis sufferers
who, like me, have been searching for a healthy
way to eliminate this stubborn, embarrassing
and irritating skin condition
while attempting to maintain a healthy sex life.

GW00645318

CHAPTER 1
SHIT HAPPENS!

"It" appeared in the form of a moon-shaped mark at the bottom of my hairline after a five-hour flight from San Diego to Boston. I blamed it on something I must have picked up off the headrest during the flight. It was red and itchy and ran from ear to ear across the back of my neck.

This was the beginning of a disease that would mark my once "perfect skin" for the next twenty-five years.

An article in a women's fashion magazine stated;

"The number one attraction between lovers is their skin."

Oh dear! I was in serious trouble. Over the next two decades I watched with horror as my silky soft skin slowly turned into a crumbled maze of scaly, flaky patches. As my skin deteriorated so did my pride, confidence and sexual relationships. My glorious sexual freedom of the past slowly slipped into an embarrassment of covered limbs and "lights off" moments shared in darkness and deceit.

Psoriasis

The Simple Cure
Who knew?

Leonie Mateer

Psoriasis – The Simple Cure -Who Knew?
Copyright © 2016 by Leonie Mateer. All rights reserved

The information in this book is based solely on the opinion and experience obtained by the author who has been a psoriasis sufferer for over twenty-five years. It is in no way meant to be a medical guide and the author advises that any change to your diet should be discussed with your medical practitioner or practiced individual.

Published in the United States of America

1. Non Fiction: Health/Wellness
2. General Non Fiction – Health/Diet/Wellness

1/5/17

ISBN 13 9780997657463

I had just turned forty when psoriasis entered my daily existence.

I was a successful entrepreneur at the top of my game, living the American dream and thought this annoying skin disease could be conquered and beaten. After all, I could control every other aspect of my life, why should a skin problem be any different?

A twenty-five year journey of living with psoriasis, researching cures, applying ointments, taking recommended medications and changing my eating habits has inspired me to write this book.

I do realize psoriasis is personal to every individual. What works for me may not work for you. However, by sharing my experiences and what I have learned during the process of attempting to eliminate this horrible disfiguring disease, I hope my story can offer you some solace in your own journey.

CHAPTER 2
TAR, ROMANCE AND MAGIC

The first few years were almost bearable with patches appearing on my elbows, knees, hairline and tummy. The tummy was the worse. A two-inch circular patch sat just above my bikini line caused me extreme embarrassment during sex. This was in the early nineties and I had tried the nasty smelling coal tar treatments and various vitamin D ointments with little or no success.

Coal tar. A thick, black byproduct of the manufacture of petroleum products and coal, coal tar is probably the oldest treatment for psoriasis. It reduces scaling, itching and inflammation. Exactly how it works isn't known. Coal tar has few known side effects, **but it's messy, stains clothing and bedding, and has a strong odor.**

Vitamin D analogues. These synthetic forms of vitamin D slow down the growth of skin cells. Calcipotriene **(Dovonex)** *is a prescription cream or solution containing a vitamin D analogue that may be used alone to treat mild to moderate psoriasis or in combination with other topical medications or phototherapy. This treatment can irritate the skin. Calcitriol (Rocaltrol) is expensive but may be equally effective and possibly less irritating than calcipotriene.* **I use Daivonex – have done so for as long as I can remember. It softens the plaques. Once the tube has been open for a while it** *is less effective. A new tube always gives the best results. As it contains no steroids it is an ideal everyday product.*

I was on a romantic getaway in New Zealand with a kiwi lover at the time and had read somewhere, if you rub a white quartz crystal on the infected area and then throw the quartz into the ocean, your psoriasis patch will completely disappear.

I was desperate and prepared to try anything.

We were staying in a romantic little cottage on a desolate beach. Early one morning I sneaked out of bed and made my way down to the water's edge carrying my precious white quartz crystal full of hope and expectation. I lay on the warm summer sand and, with closed eyes; I rubbed my "spot" with complete concentration – willing it to disappear. Finally I walked towards the lapping waves of the ocean with crystal in hand feeling rather foolish at what I was about to do.

The crystal was quite large and expensive so frugally I decided to throw it close to shore hoping to retrieve it once the magic had activated. But alas within moments it was gone. I searched and searched but the sand and sea had surreptitiously claimed it so I returned to the cottage and my sleeping lover feeling cheated and ridiculous.

Upon my return to the States I continued faithfully to apply my Daivonex ointment on the troublesome patch while lying in the Californian sunshine and, within a couple of weeks, the patch completely disappeared – gone - never to return again. Strangely every other patch, not magically rubbed with quartz and thrown into the ocean, continued to exist no matter how long I rubbed with ointment and exposed them to the sun. I often wondered about the disappearing magical patch. I also wondered why I didn't purchase multiple quartz (one for every patch) and attempt this magical cure again. I never did.

During those early years I rubbed on ointments to keep the affected patches moist. By evening they were dry and flaky requiring me to repeat the process before climbing into bed with my lover. It was imperative the dry plaques could not be "felt" in the dark.

I was living daily with the shame of a skin disease.

Little did I know the patches would grow and my body would eventually be covered over seventy-five percent with what I had become to despise – my shitty psoriasis.

The years took on a daily ritual. Soak in the bath, moisten patches with ointments in the morning and repeat the process in the evening before bed.

The patches were multiplying silently and steadily.

My fingers knew where the patches were without looking. Applying the ointment was ritualistic. If I waited too long after leaving the bath or shower, the patches would thicken and dry. Its importance became paramount. It also had to be done in complete secret. I kept tubes of Daivonex ointment in the bathroom and in the bedroom – hidden in drawers and cupboards.

It was my secret, my embarrassment, and my Achilles heel.

CHAPTER 3
FALSE HOPE AND A DIRE DATE.

One day I was talking to a neurologist who told me his dermatologist injected a steroid solution into his plaque areas eliminating them completely. He only had a couple of spots on his scalp. The Doctor warned me it was only a temporary solution and needed to be repeated every few months. I was so excited and immediately made an appointment with his dermatologist who obliged, upon my request, to inject my patches one by one with a steroid solution. At this time my psoriasis was mostly on my knees, elbows, neck and scalp. I had lost a lot of weight and my body was looking in the best shape it had looked for many years. If only I could clear my skin of psoriasis.

To my amazement my psoriasis completely disappeared. It was a miracle. Within a couple of weeks I was single, slim and, for the first time in years, I had a clear skin. It was wonderful!

To celebrate my newly gained psoriasis freedom I invited my new boyfriend to share a glass of champagne and "hors d'oeuvres" on my balcony overlooking Hollywood Beach. We drank and laughed in the warm breezy night air. We watched the sunset and dipped fresh shrimp into red wet sauces. After too many glasses of champagne and a false sense of bravery I took his hand and led him up the stairs to my big king size bed.

So many years of hiding my scarred body were suddenly replaced with the courage to remove my clothing and stand naked in full light exposing my perfectly tanned, clear skin in all its beauty.

My date lay in between the sheets wondering, I am sure, at my rather strange behavior and beckoned me to join him in bed. I did. Happy and free. I turned towards him expecting him to be in awe of my sheer beauty.

He clutched at his chest and asked me if I had any Aspirin. I didn't. I offered Excedrin - which he said was full of caffeine and would not do.

Redressed he headed down the stairs and out the front door to his truck in the driveway. Confused and rejected, I followed his lead, meeting him, upon his return, lying on my dining room floor begging me to find a doctor *"now!"*

Having just moved to Oxnard from Santa Barbara and completely intoxicated from excess champagne I began to search for medical doctors in my Santa Barbara phone book. The words were blurry and I had no idea what urgent care facility was close by. The man yelled between gasps. "We are not in Santa Barbara, call 999. " I did.

Within two minutes a room full of dashing men in fire fighting gear stood in my dining room. They whisked my date away on a stretcher. I was told to follow the ambulance in my car. What ambulance? I listened to the siren disappearing into the night. I walked around in circles, confused, disoriented, alarmed, disappointed, horrified. *What had I done?*

Too drunk to drive but not drunk enough to know better, I grabbed my keys and headed out the door to the hospital where I sat anxiously in the empty waiting room. I checked the time. It was two in the morning. I waited and waited until finally a man in white coat asked me if I was with "the man with the heart condition." I followed him through cold corridors to a room with half a dozen nurses and doctors surrounding my date - my date who was obviously at death's door.

When he saw me he gasped, "She nearly killed me!" Was he joking? How could he joke?

The doctor said, "We cannot operate until his condition improves. Does he have family? His condition is serious. Family? I don't even remember his last name! "He has a brother, I think?" I racked my brain to remember a previous conversation. I realized this man was a stranger. I shook my date until his eyes focused on me. "What's your brother's phone number?"

He couldn't respond. He was dying. It was my fault! I must have scared the living daylights out of him. He was a shy man - a marathon runner, so healthy and fit. How could he possibly be the one having the heart attack?

Our fourth date was in the hospital while I held his arm and did "slow walkies" up and down the corridor. I felt responsible, guilty.

I was due to leave for New Zealand the next week to visit my newly built dream home on a rural hill overlooking a magnificent harbour. The man could not return to work. He needed to recuperate. The operation had gone well. He had over ninety per cent blockages in his arteries. He had almost died.

Two weeks we spent in New Zealand. It was my fiftieth birthday. I was still psoriasis free, slender and happy.

On my birthday night I ran a bath in my new air bath surrounded by marble and bubbling with bath balls and fragrance. I lay seductively enticing my male guest to join me. He blamed his weak condition and chose instead to sweep the floor and tidy the room. It was not a successful holiday.

Upon our return, I bade him farewell. Later I heard he had married a French copywriter and was blissfully happy.

Being psoriasis free turned out to be just a short window in time.

I knew it was a quick fix and not a healthy choice. My psoriasis returned with a vengeance (too severe to repeat the same treatment) and I was left with the memory of what it felt like to be psoriasis free. Only psoriasis sufferers can relate to the miracle of a few precious weeks with clear skin. I never forgot what it felt like. It would take many more years before I would discover the cause of the disease and eventually have clear skin for life.

CHAPTER 4:
DRUGS, DRUGS AND MORE DRUGS.

Patches on elbows and knees are bearable and easy to disguise. Three quarter sleeve tops and jeans and tights can easily hide your disfigurement.

But by the time I was in my late fifties, my psoriasis had become a nightmare.

My upper thighs, lower legs, upper and lower back, buttocks, under my breasts, my forearms, upper arms, knees, elbows and stomach were so deeply affected my social life and sex life had become almost impossible.

After ten years of dating I finally settled into a long-term relationship and hid my disfigurement during the day and suffered with makeshift disguises during the night.

Tubes of Daivonex sat hidden in my bedside drawer, bathroom cabinet, and dresser drawers. Constant baths and a body slimy with ointments were my norm. My little grandchildren began to notice that the arms of the dining room chairs were slippery and their "Bubba" left little white flakes on the sofa and on her bedroom floor.

Shoulders speckled with white flecks marred my dark business attire and exposed my secret on a daily basis.

It never stopped. I was constantly brushing away my humiliation and living in denial that one day I would be healed.

In desperation I again researched my options. Advertisements appeared on television for a cure. Humira, Stelara, Enbrel. Movie stars and models were being cleared of their plaque psoriasis. Was it a dream come true?

What was worse, I now suffered from psoriatic arthritis. I went to my doctor who at first couldn't explain the sudden pain and weakness in one ankle until a few months later both ankles were affected. I was immediately referred to a rheumatologist. I constantly limped and, at times, I tumbled to the ground when my ankles simply "gave way". I was in trouble.

I was shocked to read that up to thirty percent of people with psoriasis also develop psoriatic arthritis.

Psoriatic Arthritis (PSA) causes pain, stiffness and swelling around the joints and typically affects the ankle, knees, fingers, toes and lower back. Oh, lucky me.

If having a body covered in scales was not bad enough, now I worried I would not be able to walk without pain again.

Around this time I was writing my new novel series in New Zealand and made an appointment with a local dermatologist to request the marvel drug – Stelara.

The Doctor was kind, even sympathetic. I qualified, he said.

I had the required seventy five percent of my body affected by psoriasis.

But before he could legally prescribe Enbrel or Stelara I had to first try oral medication. Damn! I left that day with the first of many oral prescriptions. Methotrexate and, later Neoral Cyclosporine. My lips swelled, my gums bled, my hair fell out and my body rejected the medications with vigor.

I had already tried Daivobet ointment with no success as my body had reacted adversely to the steroid ingredient.

Daivobet 50/500 Gel (psoriasis, eczema and other scaly skin treatments (retinoid and topical medicines)) is a brand of medicine containing the active ingredients; Calcipotriol – betamethasone dipropionate (psoriasis, eczema and other scaly skin treatments (retinoid and topical medicines)) is an active ingredient that is used in some medicines.

*Retinoids. Related to vitamin A, this group of drugs may reduce the production of skin cells if you have severe psoriasis that doesn't respond to other therapies. Signs and symptoms usually return once therapy is discontinued, however. Side effects may **include lip inflammation and hair loss**. And because retinoids such as acitretin (Soriatane) can cause severe birth defects, women must avoid pregnancy for at least three years after taking the medication.*

*Methotrexate. Taken orally, methotrexate helps psoriasis by decreasing the production of skin cells and suppressing inflammation. It may also slow the progression of psoriatic arthritis in some people. Methotrexate is generally well tolerated in low doses but may cause upset stomach, loss of appetite and fatigue. When used for long periods, it can cause **a number of serious side effects,** including severe liver damage and decreased production of red and white blood cells and platelets.*

Finally, after exhausting all the oral medication options I knew I would now be approved for Enbrel.

I attended my next appointment expecting to receive a prescription and instructions on how to inject the drug into my body in the hope that my psoriasis would finally be controlled. Enbrel, here I come!

Enbrel, Humira and Selara
*Drugs that alter the immune system (biologics). Several immunomodulator drugs are approved for the treatment of moderate to severe psoriasis. They include etanercept (**Enbrel**), infliximab (Remicade), adalimumab (**Humira**) and ustekinumab (**Stelara**). These drugs are given by intravenous infusion, intramuscular injection or subcutaneous injection and are usually used for people who have failed to respond to traditional therapy or who have associated psoriatic arthritis. Biologics work by blocking interactions between certain immune system cells and particular inflammatory pathways. Although they're derived from natural sources rather than chemical ones, they must be used with caution because they have strong effects on the immune system and may permit life-threatening infections. In particular, people taking these treatments must be screened for tuberculosis.*

My dreams were shattered when my doctor advised me that because my family has a history of MS, I did not qualify for the drug, after all. My six months of taking oral medication had only worsened my condition.

My options now were reduced to a tube of Daivonex and a lifetime of embarrassment and disfigurement. I was devastated.

I agreed to visit the doctor again in a few months. Hopefully he'd have an alternative option for me.

I wasn't holding my breath.

CHAPTER 5
WHO KNEW?

My two daughters live in the USA. I brought them to the USA when they were pre-teens. Junior high, high school, university and careers kept them there. They married American born husbands and gave birth to American born boys – two each. Hence I have lived half my life in New Zealand and half in the United States of America.

My life took an unexpected turn when, almost two years ago, I took one of many trips from California to Auckland on Air New Zealand.

On board I watched the movie *"That Sugar Film"* and it finally gave me hope.

THAT SUGAR FILM is one man's journey to discover the bitter truth about sugar. Damon Gameau embarks on a unique experiment to document the effects of a high sugar diet on a healthy body, consuming only foods that are commonly perceived as 'healthy'. Through this entertaining and informative journey, Damon highlights some of the issues that plague the sugar industry, and where sugar lurks on supermarket shelves. THAT SUGAR FILM will forever change the way you think about 'healthy' food.

Further reading on diets led me to another amazing fact –

Psoriasis lives in an acidic body!

Was my body acidic? I purchased a packet of pH test strips and, sure enough, my body was completely acidic. Who knew? It was a revelation. Why hadn't anyone told me about this? Now I could finally do something myself. I would transform my body into an alkaline state and rid myself of this awful disease. It was my last hope. I had tried everything else. Nothing had worked. Even the early steroid injections into my infected areas that gave me a few months of temporary relief could no longer be used. My psoriasis was too severe and too widespread. Plus I never found another dermatologist who even agreed to do this treatment.

I immediately downloaded an acid and alkaline food chart and began to change my eating habits.

Alkaline: having the properties of an alkali, or containing alkali; having a pH greater than 7.
Low pH readings (below 7.0) are considered acidic, while higher readings (above 7.0) are considered alkaline. Your body functions best when the pH is slightly alkaline.

(I have included an acidic and alkaline food chart in the back of this book.)

I can just hear you say "Oh no a bloody diet!" I thought the same but I was desperate. I still felt young and vibrant but my skin and ankles looked and felt aged and weary.

Would I ever feel sexy again?

I wanted to feel proud of my body, enjoy intimacy without all the drama. So I quit sugar, dairy and followed an alkaline diet for two whole weeks! I printed out the acid/alkaline chart and stuck it to the fridge door. I watched "That Sugar Film" again and marvelled at my ignorance.

Twenty-five years I had lived with psoriasis and, more recently, with psoriatic arthritis and not one doctor had suggested I eliminate sugar, dairy and acidic foods. Why? It was so easy, so simple, and so affordable. What's more, it didn't involve toxic drugs and I could do it myself, in my home, on the road – anywhere.

Within two short weeks I could walk without pain and my psoriasis rapidly began to heal.

From my alkaline food chart I learned about Rooibos tea (an alkaline tea that tastes just like black tea). I drank coconut milk and almond milk instead of cow's milk. I used olive oil spreads instead of butter. I changed to Himalayan salt -which I learned, is totally alkaline, and threw out all my other salts. I drank water with a pinch of natural baking soda (turns it alkaline). I purchased liquid chlorophyll and added it's green (from plants) liquid to my drinking water. I learned that lemons, limes and grapefruit are alkaline – not acid. Who knew?   I added parsley to my food and peppers, ginger and garlic to my stir-fry.

It worked! It's almost two years later I am still psoriasis free!

My arms, which were covered in red scaly plaque, are clear. My skin has repaired itself. My legs, for the first time in so many years are clear and healthy. My stomach is completely clear.

I began this process by eating 80% alkaline and 20% acid. Once my body had turned alkaline, I changed to 60% alkaline and 40% acid. I stopped eating sugar completely but did allow myself a couple of slices of bread each day containing a few grams of sugar.

My dermatologist was surprised and happy to see what I had achieved on my own. He confessed he had no solution to offer me medically and dreaded telling me.

"You have made my day," he said, dismissing me.

Under the New Zealand medical system I could no longer be his patient as my psoriasis was no longer 'moderate' or 'severe'. Yeah!

My ankles healed so quickly on the alkaline diet, I was amazed. Within two months all symptoms of PSA had simply disappeared.

I had a six-month wait to see a rheumatologist and by that time I almost skipped into his office on my sturdy ankles.

My rheumatologist could find no sign of psoriatic arthritis – I was completely cured!

At his request, I agreed to make a follow up appointment with his nurse in six month. At which time she examined my ankles and could find no sign of the disease. We discussed my diet and the nurse agreed with me about the negative affect sugar has on the body and confessed she was also on an alkaline diet and had lost sixty pounds and was feeling great.

When I travel, sometimes I make bad

food choices then my psoriasis returns in a very mild form. Quickly, I revert to 80/20 alkaline/acid diet and, weather permitting; I spend fifteen minutes of sun exposure daily. I have always used Daivonex (Vitamin D Cream/Ointment) to enhance the effect of the sun on my psoriasis patches.

If natural sun is not an option, I use a sunbed fifteen minutes a day for a couple of weeks until my skin clears.

Sun Bed Treatment:
Most tanning beds deliver only UVA light, which does not treat psoriasis, so you need a tanning bed that provides both UVB and UVA light

As I write this book for you, I am at my sister's house in London. She also suffers from psoriasis and has since her mid forties. Her daughter, whom I haven't seen for almost seven years, said my skin looks wonderful. I look younger and healthier than I did when she last saw me.

My skin glows, I am glowing. To finally be free of psoriasis is sheer happiness! In the end, it was so simple. Who knew?

It's worth it!

Try going sugar free, dairy free and stick to an 80/20 alkaline/acid diet for a few weeks and see if you get the same results. I really hope you do. Let me know. I would love to hear from you. If you have a few white quartz crystals lying about, you might want to give that a go too. You never know.

I wish you beautiful clear skin, a healthy glow and a psoriasis free future.

DIETARY NOTES

How to alkaline your water: (four options)

Drink at least four large glasses of water a day.

* Add **baking soda.** Add 1/8 tbsp. (600 mg) baking (bicarbonate) soda to an 8 oz. (0.237 liters) glass of water. Purchase your baking soda from any health food shop.

* Add **lemon juice.** Lemons are anionic, so when you drink water with lemon juice added, your body reacts with the anionic properties of the lemon making the water alkaline as your body digests it. ... Use only fresh lemons – just a squeeze or two per glass.

* Add **Liquid Chlorophyll** to your water. I use Liquid Chlorophyll drops from Benevolent Nourishment – 15 drops added to each glass of drinking water.

* Add **pH drops.**
pH drops are a powerful solution which - when added to drinking water - raise the pH of that water.

Note: For quick results I have found that using Liquid Chlorophyll drops or liquid Chlorophyll concentrate added to my drinking water is the most effective.

But, like everything you eat, variety is the spice of life, so change at leisure your alkaline water options – I do.

Test your pH Balance on a regular basis to ensure you are in the perfect zone

The ideal pH is slightly alkaline - 7.30 to 7.45. You can test your pH levels regularly by using a piece of litmus paper in your saliva or urine first thing in the morning before eating or drinking anything.

You can purchase **pH test strips** for saliva or urine online at Amazon or other health food outlets.

A pH less than 7 is said to be acidic and solutions with a pH greater than 7 are basic or alkaline.

ALKALINE/ACIDIC CHART

Highly Alkaline

pH 9.5 alkaline water
(See page 26 for details on how to alkaline your
water)

Himalayan Pink Salt
(This is a must – the only salt I now use)

Grasses
Cucumber
Kale
Kelp
Spinach
Parsley
Broccoli
Sprouts (soy, alfalfa etc.)
Sea Vegetables (Kelp)
Green drinks
All Sprouted Beans/ Sprouts

Moderately Alkaline
Avocado
Beetroot
Capsicum/Pepper
Cabbage
Celery
Collard/Spring Greens
Endive
Garlic
Ginger
Green Beans
Lettuce
Mustard Greens
Okra
Onion
Radish
Red Onion
Rocket/Arugula
Tomato

Lemon
Lime

Butter Beans
Soy Beans
White Haricot Beans
Chia/Salba
 Quinoa

Mildly Alkaline

Artichokes
Asparagus
Brussels Sprouts
Cauliflower
Carrot
Chives
Courgette/Zucchini
Leeks
New Baby Potatoes
Peas
Rhubarb
Swede
Watercress
Grapefruit
Coconut
Buckwheat
Quinoa
Spelt
Lentils
Tofu
Other Beans & Legumes
Goat & Almond Milk
Most Herbs & Spices
Avocado Oil
Coconut Oil
Flax Oil/ Udo's Oil

Neutral/Mildly Acidic

Black Beans
Chickpeas/Garbanzos
Kidney Beans
Seitan

Cantaloupe
Currants
Fresh Dates
Nectarine
Plum
Sweet Cherry
Watermelon

Amaranth
Millet Oats/Oatmeal
Spelt
Soybeans
Rice/Soy/Hemp Protein

Freshwater Wild Fish
Rice & Soy Milk

Brazil Nuts
Pecan Nuts
Hazel Nuts
Sunflower Oil
Grape seed Oil

Moderately Acidic

Fresh, Natural Juice
Ketchup
Mayonnaise
Butter
Apple
Apricot
Banana
Blackberry
Blueberry
Cranberry
Grapes
Mango
Mangosteen
Orange
Peach
Papaya
Pineapple
Strawberry
Brown Rice
Oats
Rye Bread
Wheat
Wholemeal Bread
Wild Rice
Wholemeal
Pasta

Ocean Fish

Highly Acidic

Alcohol
Coffee & Black Tea
Fruit Juice (Sweetened)
Cocoa
Honey
Jam
Jelly
Mustard
Miso
Rice Syrup
Soy Sauce
Vinegar
Yeast
Dried Fruit
Beef
Chicken
Eggs
Farmed Fish
Pork
Shellfish
Cheese
Dairy
Artificial Sweeteners
Syrup
Mushroom

Drug information obtained by:
http://www.mayoclinic.org/diseases-
conditions/psoriasis/basics/treatment/con-20030838

That Sugar Film
www.thatsugarfilm.com
Filmmaker Damon Gameau documents the effects of
eating supposedly healthy foods that contain high
amounts of sugar.
Initial Release February 2015 (Australia)
Also available in book form "That Sugar Book"

Acid and Alkaline Food Charts:
https://liveenergized.com/
Ross Bridgeford is a writer, health coach and nutrition
addict & his dream is to ENERGIZE the World.
        This dream started in 2004 with the creation of
energiseforlife.com, where he has published over 600
guides, recipes and articles, read by over 2 million
people every year.
        Ross is the author of two Alkaline Diet Recipe
Books and the Amazon best seller "The Water Diet".
        Ross has also coached thousands of clients to
their dream health through his courses: The Alkaline
Diet Course, The Alkaline Weight Loss Solution & the
Alkaline Cleanse Program.

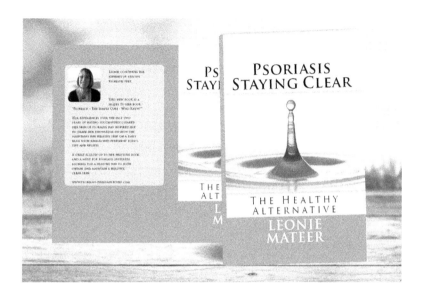

Leonie Mateer continues her journey of staying psoriasis free with her new book "Psoriasis -Staying Clear. The Healthy Alternative."

Her experience over the past two years and a half years of having successfully cleared her skin of psoriasis has inspired her to share her knowledge of how she maintains her healthy skin on a daily basis with pertinent researched topics, tips, blogs and recipes.

A great follow-up to her previous successful book "Psoriasis - The Simple Cure -Who Knew? And a must read or all psoriasis sufferers looking for a healthy way to obtain and maintain clear skin.

A comprehensive collection of her "tried and true" healthy recommendations for clearing psoriasis include:

- Psoriasis – Before and After
- The "No No'" List of Acidic Foods
- How to test your pH levels
- Baking Soda and Psoriasis
- Moisturize for clear, healthy skin
- Liquid Chlorophyll – the green healer
- Traveling with Psoriasis
- 10 Best Tips for Healing Psoriasis
- Psoriasis Foods – What Heals?
-

And much more….

The information in this book is also available on the website: www.psoriasis-thesimplecure.com/blog

ABOUT THE AUTHOR

Leonie Mateer was born and raised in New Zealand, but moved to the United States in her 30s to pursue business opportunities. She lived back in New Zealand for several years in the 2000s, running a luxury lodge in Northland, and now splits her time between New Zealand and the USA.

Mateer is known as a brand development expert and has previously written business advice books.

PSORIASIS – THE SIMPLE CURE -WHO KNEW?
her first health and wellness book is followed by PSORIASIS – STAYING CLEAR – THE HEALTHY ALTERNATIVE

She has also written THE AUDREY MURDERS – a five book thriller series, starring Audrey, a serial killer living in idyllic small-town New Zealand. Other books include: THE MAGICAL WORLD OF DANTONIA (mid-grade), BLACK LAKE (mid-grade), THE BIRD BOYS (mid-grade) and THE CABOODLES BLUEPRINT (business advise)

Website: www.psoriasis-thesimplecure.com
www.leoniemateer.com
Email: **leoniemateer@yahoo.com**

If you have found this book helpful, I would love you to leave a review on Amazon.

Happy healing.
Leonie Mateer